HOW MY IMMUNE SYSTEM BEAT CANCER

Fasting, Juicing, Ketogenic diet, Breathing, Exercise, Meditation and other non-toxic therapies

> "*May food be thy medicine.*"
> — Hippocrates

> *"When diet is wrong, medicine is of no use. When diet is right, medicine is of no use."*
>
> - Old Ayurveda proverb

"Fred is a patient of mine and a close friend, and I wrote the foreword for this book. I can personally guarantee the reality of his incredible healing. A reality confirmed by MRIs and bloodwork. We live in a time of "one problem, one pill" and Fred's adventure is an incredible testimony that things could be different."

- Dr. Charles Gibert

TABLE OF CONTENTS

Forewords

Warning

Introduction

Part 1: My story

Part 2: What I've learned

Part 3: My protocol

Part 4: Keto recipes

Conclusion

Appendix

Bibliography

Resources for further research

About the author

Not incurable but in-curable
(curable from within)

1ˢᵗ **Foreword** by Doctor Charles Gibert

If curing cancer using mostly natural methods seems too good to be true, it's because we don't ask the right questions. First, we need to truly understand what cancer is telling us.

Here is an analogy: if a light comes on, on your car's dashboard because of a malfunction, would you ignore it? Illness **is** that light. If that signal is not followed by an attentive dialogue with your own body; if you do not accept to find new and appropriate answers to your body's problems, then all the lights on the dashboard will eventually turn on, and then things will get a lot more complicated and difficult to repair.

Imagine a radio program, where the "Who's Who" of Energy, Body and Soul were invited: "And the word was made flesh", Jesus would say, quoting the Bible; "Matter is a manifestation of energy" would add Einstein; "Yes, everything is energy" would say Lao Tsu, quoting the Dao De Ching. And Hippocrates would bring everyone together by calmly saying: "Cancer is a manifestation of energy." Freud, who just arrived, would add "but Cancer is also a manifestation of emotion."

All stress, physical or psychological, induces an accumulation of energy which, when it becomes chronic, automatically leads to some physical manifestation.

Energy, time and matter, from Einstein's famous equation, are also involved in the equations of psychosomatic medicine. Those who have understood this, no longer treat diseases according to conventional treatments only.

Those who have understood this, take a new approach to healing. When they talk about Energy, they talk about its circulation and its physical or psychological blockages. Those people begin to dream that what has been tied up in a tumor can be untied with a natural cure. And they are right!

One of those people is my friend, Fred Evrard, and he did it.

2nd **Foreword** by Lila Evrard

The day Fred was diagnosed with cancer, my whole world collapsed. We always believed that this couldn't happen to us because of our healthy life-style! I remember I was at home in the US with only my puppy, while Fred was in France for medical exams - for what we thought was only an intestinal inflammation. He called me to tell me that the doctors said it was cancer, and it was already stage 3. I broke in tears.

The doctors said that looking at his family's cancer history and the advance stage of his cancer, he would probably be dead already if not for his healthy lifestyle and ketogenic diet. When something like that happens in your life, it puts everything else in perspectives. Cancer becomes your whole world. Since I've known him (we've been married for 18 years), Fred was always so strong and so brave... He fought so many battles in his life, but I knew that this one would be the hardest of them all.

We can't realize how difficult it is until you are in the middle of it. I saw him in so much pain; I still don't know how he did it. But I knew he would fight for his life; for me, for his family, for his students, no matter how hard.

Now, less than 4 months after the beginning of his natural healing, Fred is completely cured! I believe his 'experience' is unique because he used many different holistic tools to reach this goal and he faithfully believed that his immune system and his "warrior" mental strength could heal him more surely that any chemical and toxic treatment. I encouraged him to share his journey by writing a book, this book, as I truly believe it can help a lot of people.

Living with Fred in our house in South Carolina, and having been a direct witness of how well and fast he beat this cancer, using the traditional knowledge of fasting, nutrition, Tai Chi, meditation, etc., and refusing the heavy long-term chemotherapy, radiation and surgery oncologists told him he had to do to survive, I can say that I have never been so proud of him. He showed me, and everyone we know, what true courage is.

You see, there is more than one path to treat cancer (and any disease for that matter) and we too often think the only way is through chemotherapy, radiation and surgery. We chose to go more towards the natural path (holistic medicine, traditional Chinese medicine, nutrition, fasting...). That's exactly what Fred will be sharing with you in this book. How his immune system beat cancer!

I am so proud of him to have fought this ultimate battle so bravely and fearlessly.

I saw so many cancer patients going through hell during our few visits at the hospital, I wished all of them knew what to do to heal naturally; working with their body and immune system and not against them, without those horrible side effects from chemo and radiation.

Fred wrote this book from his personal experience and from the research he did during those difficult times. We have always taught by example and from experience (we both have been teaching martial arts and health for more than 30 years), and this will validate everything we believe in and teach, and hopefully help a lot of people.

Positivity and mental strength are also super important. No matter how hard life is and what it brings us, we must always remember what one of our masters reminded us one day, in Baisha, China, during our 4-year trip around the world: DON'T WORRY, BE HAPPY!*

Our body has all the keys to heal; work with it, not against it!

*Doctor Ho: Famous traditional Chinese medicine doctor in Yunnan province, China.

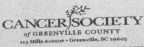

CANCER SOCIETY
of GREENVILLE COUNTY
113 Mills Avenue • Greenville, SC 29605

PHYSICIAN'S STATEMENT

__Frederic Evrard__ is receiving services provided by the Cancer Society of Greenville County.

THE PATIENT/GUARDIAN, BY SIGNING BELOW, HEREBY GIVES PERMISSION TO HIS/HER PHYSICIAN TO RELEASE THE HEALTH INFORMATION LISTED BELOW:

Patient or Guardian's Signature ▓▓▓▓▓▓▓▓▓▓▓▓▓▓

Date of Birth 10-13-72

▓▓▓▓▓▓▓▓▓▓▓▓▓▓

Date 11-5-20

City ▓▓▓▓▓ State Zip   Phone

THE *CANCER* PHYSICIAN SHOULD COMPLETE THE FOLLOWING AND MAIL TO THE ABOVE ADDRESS, OR FAX TO THE NUMBER BELOW:

Patient: __Frederic Evrard__

Diagnosis: __Rectal CA__   (NO CODES, PLEASE)

Prognosis: __Stable__

CANCER RELATED DRUGS **ONLY**: _____

Comments: _____

*Should patient receive nutritional supplements due to cancer-related causes?__ yes__

*Does patient require disposables (diapers, pads, etc.) due to cancer-related causes?_____

Physician's Signature

__900 W. Fans Rd__
Address

__Greenville SC 29605__
City   State   Zip

Phone __404-2010__

Date __11-6-20__

3/3/2016

Phone (864) 232-8439 • Fax (864) 232-7311 • E-mail info@cancersocietygc.org • Website www.cancersocietygc.org

PRISMA

HEALTH.

10/15/2020

To Whom It May Concern:

 Frederic Aime Evrard was in my office on 10/12/2020.He is being treated by my office for adenocarcinoma, rectal cancer. He will be undergoing chemo and then chemo radiation. He will possibly undergo surgery after this treatment and then continue treatment post op. During this time he may become weak and require a care giver full time to provide assistance in daily living activities as well as emotional support related to cancer diagnosis and treatment.

If you have questions or concerns, please don't hesitate to call our office at 864-699-5700.

Sincerely,

███████████, MD
CANCER INSTITUTE MDC
890 W. FARIS ROAD, STE 320
GREENVILLE SC 29605-4281
864-455-1200

The hospital in South Carolina confirmed the diagnostic and proposed treatment from the hospital in France

10/17/20 MRI Study Result
Mr. Frederic Evrard – Oct. 13, 1972

Impression

Evidence of near circumferential tumor involving the distal rectum and proximal anus with similar irregular thickening of the involved segment of the rectum.

Slice by slice comparison of the axial thin section images document more heterogeneous T2 signal intensity throughout the involved mucosal/submucosa but thickness, distribution, and contours remain similar to previous exam.

Stable mesorectal nodes.

Signed by: 10/17/2020: M███ S██████, MD

Narrative

EXAM: MRI RECTUM WO CONTRAST, 10/17/2020

INDICATION: C20 Malignant neoplasm of rectum I10;

TECHNIQUE: Multiplanar/multisequence pelvic MRI performed without IV contrast including thin section angled axial and coronal images, oriented to the distal rectal tumor.

FINDINGS:

Distortion of the distal rectum related to treated 75% circumference tumor involving the distal rectum and proximal anus. Approximately 6 to 7 cm in length and terminates approximately 1.8 cm from the anal verge.

1/10/21 MRI Study Result
Mr. Frederic Evrard – Oct. 13, 1972

Impression

No more evidence of circumferential tumor involving the distal rectum and proximal anus

Signed by: 1/10/2021: M███ S█████ MD

Narrative

EXAM: MRI RECTUM WO CONTRAST, 01/10/2021

INDICATION:

COMPARISON: Pelvic MRI 9/17/2020.

TECHNIQUE: Multiplanar pelvic MRI without contrast. This includes thin section angled axial and coronal images, oriented to the distal rectal tumor.

FINDINGS:

No more evidence of circumferential tumor involving the distal rectum and proximal anus. No interval local progression of disease is observed. No new adenopathy elsewhere in the pelvis.

14

Warning

Dear reader,

Please note that I am not a doctor. I am not trying to convince you of anything and I am not encouraging you to make changes for which you might not be ready. All I wanted to achieve with this book was to share my experience of healing from cancer naturally, and to highlight the doctors and people who can think outside of the box when talking about cancer treatments and therapies. Doctor Charles Gibert, Doctor Nasha Winters, Doctor Valter Longo, Doctor Eric Berg, Professor Thomas Seyfried, Doctor Jean-Pierre Lablanchy, Thierry Casasnovas and Professor Henry Joyeux's works were a big part of my journey and their books not only inspired me, but also gave me the scientific knowledge I needed to better understand what my intuition and 40-year of experience in martial arts and Asian medicines taught me: Remove the cause and the symptom disappears.

We have become a pro-cancer society and our environment (internal and external) is both the cause of diseases and the key to our health. Most of what industrials sell us is carcinogenic, from the toxic processed food and food-by products, pesticides, food preservatives, antibiotics in our meat, plastic particles in our water, mercury in our fish, air, water and soils pollution, stress, lack of physical activities, toxic relationships, over consumption of medical drugs, over-vaccinations, hours of seating in front of a screen, and much more... Yes, we have become a sick and pro-cancer society. But the good news is, it is easy to make just a few changes to improve our health and our lives.

Last clarification: not having really planned to write a book when I was at my worst, I did not keep a "diary". It is therefore possible that there are in this work a few errors or contradictions in terms of dates and timing. I assure you that I did my best.

I hope you will enjoy this book and that it will open the minds of cancer patients to new possibilities and hopes.

Introduction

How did a healthy guy like me get cancer? That was my first question... It was a true investigation to try to get some answers, but this journey had two positive outcomes. Number one, I survived cancer. Number two, I learned a lot about myself. 40 years of martial arts practice and 25 years teaching them, taught me how to fight... And believe me when I say this was the hardest fight of my life, both physically and mentally.

But back to my story. I grew up in a family where good and healthy food was important. Everything was fresh, my parents shopped for grocery every day, they cooked at home. We didn't eat canned food or frozen foods, the grass-fed meat came from the butcher, the vegetables from the farmers' market, the sourdough bread from the baker down the street.... Even as I grew up, I've never really had junk food, sodas, coffee, never smoked and never drank alcohol (I don't even know what it tastes like!). I started martial arts as a child and have always been interested in health, nutrition, and later, I was trained in traditional massages, acupuncture and osteopathy. I tried most of the health-oriented diets out there, such as vegetarian, vegan, raw, fasting, intermittent fasting, blood type diet, acid-alkaline balance, paleo, ketogenic, etc. In addition to martial arts, Parkour and CrossFit, I have been doing Tai Chi, Qi Gong and meditation for 30 years; I go to bed early (between 9 p.m. and 10 p.m.), I wake up early (between 5:30 a.m. and 6:30 a.m.). In short, I have always had a relatively healthy lifestyle.

But I grew up a fragile little boy. Skinny, often sick (nothing bad, but allergies every spring, cold and flu every winter and a runny nose every time two windows were open). Needless to say, I was literally fed on antibiotics and antihistamines. This didn't do well for my gut microbiome and you don't need to be a Nobel Prize to link a weak microbiome with potential colon inflammation and cancer. We also have a history of colon cancer in my family and both my father and grandfather died of it. Even though I thought I could, one doesn't run away from genetics. So, both the terrain and the genetics were already there; now, it needed a trigger... and 2020 came along!

STRESS was very probably the trigger. First, hours and hours of jetlag due to my many travels teaching martial arts all over the world, have weakened my immune system and suprarenal glands. Then, our immigration to the US, which all together cost us $100,000 and years of wait and stress. Then came covid-19, which really hurt us financially and had us closing all our Martial Arts schools around the world and cancelling all our seminars and government contracts. Finally, on September 2020, I was diagnosed with stage-3 genetic colorectum cancer. In two months, I went from the best shape of my life at 70Kg and 9% bodyfat to 49Kg of nothing but bones.

This is how it all started. After the initial shock of the diagnostic (three days of self-pity, thinking I was going to die), I raised up and had only three things in mind:

1. I'm going to survive this

2. What doesn't kill you makes you stronger

3. *"Let food be thy medicine"* (Hippocrates)

Part 1
My Journey

> "*Illnesses don't come upon us by accident. They are developed from small daily sins against Nature. When enough sins have accumulated, illness will suddenly appear*"
>
> - Hippocrates

So, on September 10, 2020, a few weeks before my 48th birthday, I was diagnosed with stage-3 genetic colon cancer. As I told you, this came as a shock because I was always convinced that my healthy lifestyle would protect me from the disease that killed both my father and my grandfather. I was wrong!

Nevertheless, it was not all for nothing, as doctors told me that without my clean and organic diet of the past 20 years and my strong athletic body, I would probably have been dead already. My life style stopped the cancer from spreading and there was no metastasis.

As for everyone in my situation, the doctors only presented me with one option (even though the odds weren't good, with only 50% chance of survival), using chemotherapy, plus radiation, plus surgery. And it was URGENT!

Against doctors' advice, I took a leap of faith and started by spending two weeks at the famous natural healing center, the *Hippocrates Health Institute* in Florida, to improve my knowledge on how fasting and raw living foods could help my body heal itself from cancer. Of course, the doctors told me that I was crazy and doomed if I didn't start chemotherapy immediately, but I was convinced otherwise and I knew I could heal naturally, without destroying my body or my immune system. And I did!

I polished and personalized my "Hippocrates protocol" based on fasting, a Ketogenic diet, anti-cancer supplements (I'll go into that later on), meditation, Tai Chi, sun exposure, deep breathing, rebounding, ice-cold bathes, psychotherapy, etc., and three weeks after starting my natural healing, the MRI showed that the tumor had shrunk from 10cm to 6cm in length and from 13mm to 5mm in depth.

The "Way of Nature" worked, yes, but it was slow (Nature takes its time) and I was in a LOT of pain. I literally spent my days and nights lying on the floor, crying, without being able to walk, sleep or even talk. I never thought my body could hurt so much. With the help of both oncologist doctors and naturopaths, I decided to do three sessions of chemo (instead of the twelve they originally wanted me to do), just for the pain, not as a treatment, and then allow my body to heal and detox from this chemical and toxic protocol. My goal was no more than three sessions of chemo, with no radiation and no surgery. It seemed impossible for my doctors, but it worked. Three sessions later, even though the cancer was still there, the pain was gone and I could go back to my natural protocol only, while living somewhat of a "normal life".

Then I continued my "custom-made" natural treatment, and exactly four months after my colonoscopy from September 10, 2020, on January 9, 2021, the tumor was completely gone.

I want to make it clear that I am not against modern medicine and certainly not against its doctors and nurses. I am fighting a system, not people. I don't think allopathic medicine is a perfect cure for cancer, but it does treat the symptoms, which is already great. For my part, I am thankful that it did help me with the pain because it was unbearable. He, who has not been there cannot know how hard it is. There were days when I wanted to die because of the pain.

But my money was on my immune system and the ability of my body to heal itself. "All" I needed to do was to minimize toxins and stress coming in and maximize the elimination and detox process. And again, I won!

The next question was **why** did my body have a need for a tumor? I believe that nothing happens by accident (even in our body). One doesn't "catch" cancer; one develops cancer, so it is created by the body. What was the physiological (or psychological) cause and how to take care of it? Simple: Less toxins in, more toxins out!

Of course, I didn't do it alone and I want to thank my doctor, nurse and healer friends without whom I couldn't have done it: Doctor Jean-Pierre Lablanchy, Doctor Charles Gibert, James Nener, Thierry Casasnovas, Sifu Amon, Delphine Beaufils, Gérard Tenque, Shannon Couch, Ari and Holly Harrison, and of course, my amazing wife Lila, my supportive mother, and so many friends, students and brothers who believed in me and my potentially dangerous decision.

THANK YOU ALL!

Part 2
What I've learned

> *"It is not because things are difficult that we do not dare; it is because we do not dare that they are difficult."*
>
> - Seneca

1.   What is cancer?

I believe that modern medicine has it wrong. Cancer is not the disease. Cancer is the symptom; an alarm that usually follows a metabolic problem, chronic inflammation, chronic fatigue or hyper-toxicity, and which tells us that there are too many wastes in our body and that our immune and lymphatic systems are too tired to fight and eliminate them properly.

Everyone develops cancer cells all the time but the body usually sheds them. Our body is designed to recognize and eliminate cells that mutate and become cancerous and it does so very effectively if it's functioning properly. So, cancer isn't the problem. The problem lies in a systemic metabolic imbalance, which results in one or more tumors that grow in the body without being stopped by the immune system. The tumor is the symptom, not the cause.

The answer to cancer is not more toxins - such as months or even years of chemotherapy and radiation (which can be useful under certain circumstances such as too much pain or too big of a tumor, but only in low doses and for a short period of time), but for me, those are certainly not the treatment. They simply help with the symptoms.

The answer is LESS toxins, more cleansing, lots of very high-quality micro and macro nutrients, lots of rest, stress management and helping the body to eliminate toxins via fasting, intermittent fasting, fasted exercise, breathing, sauna, rebounding, etc.

Here is a meta-study on the efficiency (or not) of chemotherapy for the treatment of cancer:

- I know one can find studies that say the complete opposite, and it is hard to have a clear vision of what's going on, but I prefer to trust studies that go against the pharmaceutical industry's financial benefits. -

https://pubmed.ncbi.nlm.nih.gov/15630849/

Results: *The overall contribution of curative and adjuvant cytotoxic chemotherapy to over 5-year survival in adults is estimated to be 2.3% in Australia and 2.1% in the USA.*

Conclusion: *It is clear that cytotoxic chemotherapy only makes a minor contribution to cancer survival. To justify the continued funding and availability of drugs used in cytotoxic chemotherapy, a rigorous evaluation of the cost-effectiveness and impact on quality of life is urgently required.*

2.   My method

My method is simple; it is a mix of several ancient and traditional healing systems, but the core of it is to boost the immune system, reduce inflammation, and help the body detoxify.

Liver detox:
Daily warm water with freshly squeezed lemon juice and organic apple cider vinegar
Daily sulphur-rich vegetable juices (kale, radish, garlic, beetroot...)

Boosting the immune system:
Daily Vit D3 -> 15,000 iu
Daily sun exposure
Daily Vit C -> 6 gr
Daily Vit K2 -> 200 mcg
Daily Zinc -> 30 gr
Daily cold exposure (or cryotherapy) -> outside walks at 32° (shirtless) for 20 minutes and ice-cold baths (in a river or under a waterfall) -> One to four times a week.

Reducing inflammation:
Daily Turmeric -> 3 gr
Daily Omega-3 fish oil
Daily Pre/probiotics

Elimination/cleansing:

Via the intestines -> Psyllium; colon enema (hydrotherapy); vegetable juice
Via the kidneys -> Cucumber, beetroot, parsley and celery juice
Via the skin -> sauna, dry brushing, fasting, exercise on an empty stomach (HIIT and strength training)
Via the lungs -> deep breathing
Via the lymphatic system -> rebound on a mini-trampoline, stretching

Starving the tumor:
Dry fast (24h to 36h) -> once every week
Water fast (3 days) -> once every other week
Intermittent fasting -> daily
Organic Ketogenic diet (no carbs, no sugar, no processed food) -> daily

Nourishing the body:
With food-> daily organic Ketogenic diet; fresh vegetables juices; sprouts
With breathing -> daily deep breathing (preferably outside in a natural environment)
With sun -> daily sun exposure (at least 10min. a day)
With internal energy work -> daily Chi Gong, Tai Chi or Yoga; Stretching

Stress management:
Daily meditation / prayers
Daily Tai Chi practice

Positive thinking
Laughter
Weekly Psychotherapy
Get rid of stressful environment (work, people, fear...)

3.   My top-10 anti-cancer foods

<u>All Organic of course</u>

1)   Garlic

2)   Broccoli sprouts

3)   Wheatgrass

4)   Macha green tea (infused at least 5 min.)

5)   Olive oil

6)   Fresh lemon juices

7)   Salmon, salmon roe and sardines (wild caught)

8)   Organic, pasture-raised, 100% grass-fed and grass-finished beef (meat and organ meat)

9)   Bone broth

10) Avocado

4. Five reasons why processed food is so bad for us:

1. They are engineered to be addictive with a combination of sugar, bad fats and refined white salt

2. The coloring (or bleaching) used in most processed food is very toxic

3. They are full of hazardous preservatives that have been linked to cancer

4. They are heated at very high temperature

5. Some of them are so processed that our body does not recognize them as food and literally doesn't know what to do with them

"We feed food that isn't natural to sick animals, then slaughter them to feed sick humans, who also eat food that isn't natural. This toxic system and processed carbohydrates are the root causes of a massive increase in obesity, diabetes, heart disease, cancer, neurological disease, and more."

\- Doctor Anthony Gustin

A study of over 430,000 people found that added sugar consumption was positively associated with an increased risk of esophageal cancer, pleural cancer and cancer of the small intestine.

Read the study here:

https://www.ncbi.nlm.nih.gov/pmc/articles/PMC3494407/

Another study showed that women who consumed sweet buns and cookies more than three times per week were 1.42 times more likely to develop endometrial cancer:

https://www.ncbi.nlm.nih.gov/pubmed/21765006

5.   Sugar, the real fight

From tomato sauce to most frozen dinners, added sugar can be found in even the most unexpected products. Sugar is a cheap preservative, enhances taste and is highly addictive. It is therefore the perfect "weapon" for industrials to use and make their shareholders billions of dollars. A great book by Christophe Brusset ("*Vous êtes fous d'avaler ça*" / "*You are crazy to eat that*") shows that many CEOs and traders from the food industry do not, under any circumstances, feed their family their own products.

Many people rely on quick, processed foods for meals and snacks. Since these products often contain added sugar, it makes up a large proportion of their daily calorie intake. In the US, added sugars (just sugar, not total carbs) account for up to 18% of the total calorie intake of adults and up to 15% for children. It's HUGE! Dietary guidelines suggest limiting calories from added sugar to less than 10% per day, and I believe this is still way too high for our health and optimal weight.

Most scientists and nutritionists have finally accepted that sugar consumption is a major cause of obesity and many chronic diseases, such as type-2 diabetes and type-3 diabetes (aka Alzheimer's Disease). Additionally, consuming too much sugar, especially from sugar-sweetened drinks, has been linked to atherosclerosis, a disease characterized by fatty, artery-clogging deposits.

Read the study here:

https://www.ncbi.nlm.nih.gov/pmc/articles/PMC570 8308/

Another study of over 30,000 people found that those who consumed 17–21% of calories from added sugar had a 38% greater risk of dying from heart disease, compared to those consuming only 8% of calories from added sugar:

https://www.ncbi.nlm.nih.gov/pubmed/24493081

Just one 16oz. (473mL.) can of soda contains 52gr. of sugar, which equates to more than 10% of your daily calorie consumption, based on a 2,000-calorie diet. This means that one single sugary drink a day can already put you over the recommended daily limit for added sugar.

A diet high in refined carbohydrates, including grains, sugary foods and drinks, has also been associated with a higher risk of developing skin problems such as acne, eczema and psoriasis.

Eating excessive amounts of carbs and sugar also increases your risk of developing certain cancers:

- First, a diet rich in grains, sugary foods and beverages can lead to obesity, which significantly raises your risk of cancer.

- Furthermore, diets high in carbs and sugar increase inflammation in your body and directly cause insulin resistance, both of which increase cancer risk.

A study of over 430,000 people found that added sugar consumption was positively associated with an increased risk of esophageal cancer, pleural cancer and cancer of the small intestine.

Read the study here:

https://www.ncbi.nlm.nih.gov/pmc/articles/PMC349 4407/

More research on the link between sugar and disease:

https://www.medpagetoday.com/upload/2013/3/1/j ournal.pone.0057873.pdf

https://www.ncbi.nlm.nih.gov/pubmed/19211821

https://www.sciencedirect.com/science/article/abs/ pii/0306987783900956

6. What's a Ketogenic diet?

A Ketogenic (Keto) diet simply means to switch from using glucose to using fat for fuel.

We have a rise of obesity and cancer all around the world, and it is mainly (not only) because we eat and drink too many carbohydrates, including sugar, and consume too much processed food. By cutting down carbohydrates and increasing good fat intake, we can speed up our metabolic rate, raise our HGH (Human Growth Hormone) and Testosterone levels, and lower our insulin level so we can get healthier, balance our hormones, help regenerate our cells, build muscles and burn fat at the same time. Fat also keeps you satiated much longer than carbs, so you eat less during the day. It becomes much easier to use an Intermittent Fasting protocol.

The truth is, fat is a much better and much cleaner fuel for us than glucose (basically, fat would be the equivalent of premium unleaded fuel 98 where glucose would be diesel).

The Ketogenic diet is a very low-carb, high-fat diet, which involves drastically reducing carbohydrate intake (around 30gr. per day for men and 50gr. for women) and replacing it with healthy fats. This reduction in carbs puts our body into a metabolic state called **ketosis** (the best state for our system to fight cancer by the way). When this happens, the body becomes incredibly efficient at burning fat for energy. It also turns fat into ketones in the liver, which can supply more efficient and cleaner energy for cells, including the brain.

Ketogenic diets can cause massive reductions in blood sugar and insulin levels (another good thing to fight cancer). This, along with the increased ketones, has numerous health and fitness benefits. For this reason, more and more athletes are embracing a Keto lifestyle. Once they successfully make the switch from using carbohydrates to using fats and ketones as fuel, they find themselves leaner, healthier, and more mentally focused than ever.

There are several versions of the Ketogenic diet, including:

- **Standard Ketogenic diet (SKD):** This is a 7-day a week, low-carb, moderate-protein and high-fat diet. It typically contains 70% fat, 25% protein and only 5% carbs. SKD is the most common Keto diet.

- **Cyclical Ketogenic diet (CKD):** This diet involves periods of higher-carb refeeds. I recommend once a week for athletes, and no more than once every other week for most people.

- **Targeted Ketogenic diet (TKD):** This diet allows you to have small amount of carbs during your metabolic window (around 20gr.), less than 1 hour after a workout.

- High-protein Ketogenic diet: This is similar to a standard ketogenic diet, but includes more protein. The ratio is often 55% fat, 40% protein and 5% carbs. This version of Keto is most popular among bodybuilders and strength athletes.

- Zero-carbs Ketogenic diet: This version is a high-protein and high-fat diet. It typically contains 40 to 60% fat, 60 to 40% protein and as close as possible to 0% carbs. This might be good for people with very high and chronic inflammation, and for people who have been poisoned by phytotoxins. It is the diet I used after my 21-day fast for a few months before re-introducing vegetable juices.

- Modified Keto: After the tumor was gone, I have developed my own version of the Targeted Ketogenic diet, strategically introducing root vegetable (carrot and beet) juices with a little bit of low GI fruits, on my workout days.

Foods to avoid on a Keto diet:

Any food that is high in carbohydrates should be limited. Here is a list of foods that need to be reduced or eliminated on a Keto diet:

- **Sugary foods:** Soda, fruit juice, smoothies, cake, ice cream, candy, etc.

- **Grains or starches:** Flour, bread, pasta, cereal, pastries, corn, rice, etc.

- **High GI Fruits:** Low Glycemic Index fruits such as berries (strawberries, blueberries, raspberries...), grapefruits, cherries, peaches, lemon, lime are acceptable in small quantity.

- **Beans or legumes:** Peas, peanuts, kidney beans, lentils, chickpeas, etc.

- **Root vegetables and tubers:** Potatoes, sweet potatoes, parsnips, etc. There are a few exceptions such as beets and carrots, which are not technically Keto, but are full of anti-cancer proprieties, anti-oxidants and micro-nutrients.

- **Low-fat or diet products:** These are highly processed and often high in carbs.

- **Sugar-free diet foods:** These are often high in sugar alcohols, which can affect ketone levels in some cases. These foods also tend to be highly processed. Stevia and monk-fruit are OK.

- **Some condiments or sauces:** Like ketchup or BBQ sauce... These often contain sugar and unhealthy fat.

- **Unhealthy fats:** Limit your intake of processed vegetable oils, trans fats, margarine, industrial mayonnaise, etc.

- **Alcohol:** Due to their carb content, many alcoholic beverages will throw you out of ketosis. Alcohol almost acts as sugar in the body, but with even more calories per gram.

Foods to eat on a Keto diet:

You should base the majority of your meals around these foods:

- **Seasonal vegetables:** Both green and colored. In case of colon cancer where it is better not to eat to many insoluble fibers, so juicing your veggies is the best option.

- **Butter, cream and cheese:** Preferably organic and from raw milk, grass-fed and pastured animals. If you are lactose intolerant, you can use ghee. Some people think they are lactose-intolerant but actually respond negatively to pasteurization (which is a nutritional nightmare) and to the synthetic hormones in "conventional" milk, and therefore, can digest organic raw milk cheeses perfectly well. Before we started pasteurizing our milk, dairy allergies were very rare because the (good) bacteria of the milk helped breaking down its lactose and proteins, making it easier to digest. That's why raw-milk dairy products are so much better.

- **Extra virgin organic oils, first cold pressed**: Olive oil, coconut oil and avocado oil.

- **Healthy oils:** Organic extra virgin olive oil, coconut oil, avocado oil

- **Avocados:** Whole, ripe avocados and fresh guacamole (homemade when possible).

- **Meat:** 100% grass-fed red meat, free-range chicken and turkey (organic if possible).

- **Fatty fish:** Such as salmon, trout, tuna and mackerel (wild-caught).

- **Eggs:** Look for organic pastured whole eggs. Duck eggs are great also.

- **Condiments:** You can use high quality salt (which is not supposed to be white, but grey or pink), pepper and various healthy herbs and spices.

Again, it is best to base your diet primarily on fresh, whole and organic foods. They will be much better for your health and healing.

7.   Keto diet for cancer, a metabolic disease symptom

The metabolic theory of cancer - that cancer is fueled by high carbohydrate diets - was introduced by Nobel Prize-laureate and scientist Otto Warburg in 1931. It has been largely disregarded by conventional oncology ever since, but this theory is resurging as a result of research showing incredible clinical outcomes when cancer cells are deprived of their two primary fuel sources: glucose and glutamine. YES! Food can protect us against cancer, or be a trigger for it.

"*What we have discovered is that when you to try to kill a cancer cell, one of the things it does in order to survive is to spread even further. This is why chemotherapy is not the solution*".
-    Dr. Patrick Soon-Shiong

Here is a great video by Dr. Eric Berg on how to beat cancer by removing glucose and blocking glutamine:

Cancer Lives on Sugar and... Something Else
https://www.youtube.com/watch?v=rewf0MMhGg8
&feature=youtu.be

Doctor Thomas Seyfried's work and research on the Ketogenic diet for cancer:

- Doctor Thomas Seyfried is Professor of Biology at Boston College. He is a senior editor of the American Society of Neurochemistry's journal ASN Neuro and is on the editorial boards of Journal of Lipid Research, Neurochemical Research & Nutrition & Metabolism –

Current cancer research focuses on genetic origins of cancer, and standard treatments generally involve combinations of surgery, chemotherapy and radiation. In his book "*Cancer as Metabolic Disease*", Pr. Thomas Seyfried presents an alternative origin of cancer based on the theories of Otto Warburg, wherein cancer is viewed as a disease of cellular metabolic dysfunction due to damaged mitochondria. In addition to pointing to new directions of research, Pr. Seyfried elaborates on a non-toxic mode of treatment, the ketogenic diet, which capitalizes on the inability of the damaged cancer cell mitochondria to metabolize ketones, thus starving them while maintaining healthy cells. Pr. Seyfried explains that since cancer cells ONLY feed on glucose and glutamine, using a primitive fermentation mechanism which doesn't include the use of oxygen, take away those two foods... and you cure cancer.

Here are two great interviews with Pr. Thomas N. Seyfried:

Interview with Thomas N. Seyfried on "Cancer as a Metabolic Disease"
https://www.youtube.com/watch?v=wY-JZ6TTNh8

Discussion on Cancer with Professor Thomas Seyfried - Dr Berg's Skype Interview
https://www.youtube.com/watch?v=Yyt3Do4w7fs

Doctor Nasha Winters' work and research on the Ketogenic diet for cancer:

"A 2006 University of California study found that chemotherapy causes changes to the brain's metabolism and blood flow, that can linger at least ten years after treatment. If cancer patients can survive conventional oncology's toxic treatment, they are far more likely to die earlier and with a lower quality of life. Leading cancer treatments such as chemotherapy and radiation are, in fact, carcinogenic, meaning they actually cause cancer long term. Indeed, many cancer drugs such as tamoxifen are classified by

the International Agency for Research on Cancer (IARC) as group-1 carcinogens. So is radiation"
- Dr. Nasha Winters

When cancer patients don't obtain the desired results from conventional treatments, they come to Dr. Winters as a last hope. Because of her emphasis on whole food, nutrient-dense food, a ketogenic diet and fasting, and with adequate amount of exercise, sleep, fresh water, sunlight, love and attention, she had a very different and very effective approach to preventing and neutralizing cancer for the past 25 years, including healing her own cancer (stage 4 ovarian cancer). Her approach strays significantly from conventional oncology and have been saving many lives over the years.

A new approach to cancer is sorely needed. The long-term implications of those toxic therapies can increase gut permeability, impaired cardiovascular health, depressed cognitive and neurological functions, destroy the immune system and sometimes lead to the death of the patient.

In her book *"The metabolic approach to cancer"*, she says: *"Since cancer consists of cells go awry in response of toxic diet and environments, we must optimize the body's healing mechanisms instead of waging war on them. We need to treat the terrain, not the tumor. We need to build the body up instead of attacking it. [...] When sugar, processed food, grains, soda, preservatives, additives, trans-fats, omega-6-rich oils, herbicides, pesticides and GMOs are replaced by organic vegetables and fruits, organic, 100% grass-fed meat, bone marrow and organ-meats, healthy fats and adequate hydration, the terrain shifts in a matter of days."*

Doctor Winters estimates that 90% of cancers are caused by poor, sugar-heavy diets and unhealthy lifestyles that damage mitochondrial functions.

"Cancer is not a genetic disease, as claimed by modern oncology, but instead a metabolic disorder that occurs in response to how we are feeding and treating our bodies and therefore our genomes. Through epigenetic, we have the ability to influence gene expression and mitochondrial function through our diet, lifestyle and thoughts. That's powerful medicine." she said.

Although some cancers have been proven to have a viral or bacterial origin, most of them are the result of our lifestyle, food choices and environment. Putting the patient at the core of his healing process and giving him back his responsibility for his health, rather than being a passive observer of the treatment, is the key to full and definitive recovery.

8.   Keto diet and the cholesterol myth

There is no direct relationship between fighting cancer and cholesterol, but so many people are freaking out when their cholesterol goes high on a Ketogenic diet, that it was important to straight things out concerning this urban legend.

New research is challenging the decades-old notion that saturated fat, found primarily in meat, butter and cheese, is the leading cause of clogged arteries and heart disease. The US Federal Dietary Guidelines Advisory Committee recently dropped its recommendation that healthy adults limit foods high in cholesterol, like eggs and red meat, because research shows they have very little to no effect on blood cholesterol. In fact, researchers at Yale University found that even those with coronary heart disease could safely eat up to three eggs every day for six weeks and experience no adverse effects on cholesterol levels.

Eggs are also a good source of choline, a nutrient that plays an important role in memory, and their yolk is packed with antioxidants such as lutein and zeaxanthin, which help to prevent macular degeneration.

While saturated fat does increase LDLs (wrongly called "bad" cholesterol), it increases HDLs (or "good" cholesterol) even more, keeping a very healthy ratio between the two. More and more research show that the real dietary villains are not red meat and fat but rather sugar and processed carbohydrates. They lead to more triglycerides and the formation of smaller, denser LDL particles, which in turn lead to the build-up of artery-clogging particles and inflammation by the over-reaction of mitochondria. Interestingly enough, when mitochondria burn fat for fuel, they do not cause inflammation!

A study published in 2014 in the Annals of Internal Medicine found no link between eating saturated fats and an increased risk of heart attacks. *"Foods both high and low in saturated fat can be harmful, beneficial or neutral, depending on the type of food"* says Dariush Mozaffarian, M.D., a coauthor of the study and Dean of the Friedman School of Nutrition Science and Policy at Tufts University. *"A low-carb diet, low in grains and processed foods like bread, potatoes, rice, crackers and sugar, is more effective for raising "good" cholesterol and reducing triglycerides"* he says. Adding healthy fats, such as avocados, pastured butter and extra-virgin olive oil, can also help reduce the risk of heart attack and stroke.

It is erroneous to see cholesterol as an evil, artery-clogging fat because cholesterol performs a lot of important functions in our body. It helps produce hormones, cell membranes and vitamin D, and aids in digestion. It also plays an important role in cognitive function, helping to form memories. Most of the cholesterol in your bloodstream is, in fact, created by our own body, not our diet. Our body makes 3000mg. of cholesterol per day and every cell's membrane is partially made of cholesterol. That's how important it is to us!

Read the research on cholesterol and fat myth here:

https://bmjopen.bmj.com/content/6/6/e010401.full

https://www.ncbi.nlm.nih.gov/pubmed/19082851

Another article on the same subject:

https://www.nhs.uk/news/heart-and-lungs/study-says-theres-no-link-between-cholesterol-and-heart-disease/?fbclid=IwAR3xD4i42HfRIhg5UhR6kBGQRaTex7FGzkYE0x_UgZm40lIRyGP6grioijo

Finally, hear what doctor Ken Berry has to say about the cholesterol myth:

KETO Increased Your Cholesterol? (Here's why It's OK)
https://www.youtube.com/watch?v=-QwD4xoSmRg&feature=youtu.be&fbclid=IwAR1Wq

KJio3DT2-
kEQoXunSmZB6Ut4GFSvaKkOyAwfeTS5YVJEpLrh4
MRBzQ

9.   Fasting and Intermittent Fasting

Fasting has been proven very effective for cancer prevention and cancer treatment, for both patients under chemotherapy protocol and patients following a non-toxic treatment. Also, animal studies suggest that Intermittent Fasting might prevent cancer.

Fasting and calorie restriction can slow and even stop the progression of cancer, kill cancer cells, boost the immune system, and for those who choose allopathic therapies, it can significantly improve the effectiveness of chemotherapy and radiation, and reduce the side effects.

There has been a century of research looking at the role of calorie restriction in relation to the possibility of prolonging life. While most of this research has been on animals, a modest amount of information on humans has accumulated. Specifically, risk factors for atherosclerosis and diabetes are markedly reduced in humans fasting, along with inflammatory markers, like C-reactive protein (CRP) and tumor necrosis factor (TNF).

Adaptation to starvation requires an organism to divert energy into multiple protective systems to minimize the damage that would reduce fitness. It is thought that these systems can also prolong life and decrease cancer risk. According to a review by Dr. Longo and Dr. Fontana of the University of Southern California, calorie restriction and fasting are the most powerful and reproducible physiological intervention for increasing lifespan and protecting against cancer in mammals. Fasting reduces the levels of a number of growth factors and inflammatory cytokines, reduces oxidative stress and cell proliferation, enhances autophagy (cell destruction) and several DNA repair processes.

Read different studies here:

https://osher.ucsf.edu/patient-care/integrative-medicine-resources/cancer-and-nutrition/faq/cancer-and-fasting-calorie-restriction

https://www.ncbi.nlm.nih.gov/pmc/articles/PMC2815756/

https://stm.sciencemag.org/content/4/124/124ra27.short

https://www.ncbi.nlm.nih.gov/pubmed/22323820

https://www.ncbi.nlm.nih.gov/pubmed/3245934

I personally experienced the power of fasting for healing cancer. As I mentioned above, I spent two weeks at the Hippocrates Health Institute in Florida and three weeks total fasting to save my life. One of their "tools" is feeding patients with raw living foods only (raw vegetables that is, as cancer patients are not allowed sugar, therefore no fruits). But I was in such pain and so weak that I barely ate the whole time I was there. I ate the first two days, then stopped and stayed in my room pretty much the whole time. The only nutrients I ingested were coming from a daily glass of fresh wheatgrass juice. I started to eat a little again the last four days so I basically spent two weeks on 10 calories a day (that was not hard for me as I am use to fasting and my longest was when I was in Singapore and did a three-week water fast). At the end of my retreat in Florida, I came back home to South Carolina and had my second MRI... The results were impressive and against all odds, the tumor shrunk from 10cm to 6cm in length and from 13mm to 5mm in depth without any treatment other than wheatgrass-juice fasting. I knew then that I was on the right path.

An article in US Health News mentions: "*Several studies suggest that fasting before chemo might alleviate common side effects like nausea and vomiting. There's also a growing body of research into whether fasting could have a beneficial effect against the cancer itself.*"

Two things happen when you fast. First, cancer cells can only feed on glucose (sugar) and glutamine (an amino-acid). Cut all source of those two foods and you starve the tumor. Second, when fasting, the body goes into full cleansing/elimination mode, which is the best thing you can do to remove wastes and toxins from your system. Sounds simple? Yes! but it works.

BUT if such a simple "treatment" works, why don't all the hospitals in the world use it, instead of toxic treatments? Is it possible that it's because there is no money to make from fasting patients? I don't know... but it's a valid question, knowing that the "cancer business" is worth 300 billion dollars a year. I am not against "regular" treatments, and I keep my mind open to the fact that not everyone is ready to do what I did, and that not every case needs the same solution.

Fasting also helps for chemo patients to better support the toxicity of the treatment. I personally fasted before two of my three chemo sessions, and I didn't get any of the side effects they told me I would get. No vomiting, no headaches, no diarrhea, no crash of the immune system (my immune system markers were all in normal range, which was a real surprise to the nurse who did my blood-work...). I didn't lose a single hair and I wasn't tired all the time. I wanted also to experiment not fasting before one of those three sessions (the second one), and I was sick like a dog!

Using fasting along with chemotherapy is a well-known solution and several hospitals in California, Switzerland, Germany, Turkey and Russia, use fasting to control the side effects of chemo. Usually, a 3-day fast is very effective. One day of dry fast before chemo, one day of water fast during, and one more day after that. Break the fast with coconut water or vegetable juice... Done! No side effects.

One could argue that I only did three sessions of chemo and that it might be different for patients going for the full eight to twelve sessions. Well, it's not. There are many testimonials from patients fasting during their full chemo treatment, who didn't have any side effects, or very little.

Here are two video links where Dr. Valter Longo (University of Southern California, Los Angeles) talks about his study of the positive effects of fasting on the prevention and treatment of cancer:

Extreme diets and their beneficial effects during cancer treatment
https://www.youtube.com/watch?v=1yEOJDeOM9I

Dr. Valter Longo - Fasting Cycles Retard Growth of Tumors
https://www.youtube.com/watch?v=LGafhm1cuSI

Doctor Longo says, in the second video that *"fasting is as effective or almost as effective as chemotherapy"*.

Here is another video where Tomas DeLauer, a ketogenic diet and fasting expert, presents the science behind fasting to prevent or even fight cancer:

Fasting vs. Cancer Cells: Positive Science - Thomas DeLauer
https://www.youtube.com/watch?v=WnK1FgxflWM

Here are some of the studies he used for his video:

How fasting kills cancer cells and improves immune function. (2017, May 14):

https://www.naturalhealth365.com/fasting-cancer-cells-2238.html

Fasting-like diet turns the immune system against cancer - USC News. (2018, February 5):

https://news.usc.edu/103972/fasting-like-diet-turns-the-immune-system-against-cancer/

Intermittent Fasting for Cancer Patients Mesothelioma.net.:

https://mesothelioma.net/nutrition-and-lifestyle-for-mesothelioma-patients/

Is there a role for carbohydrate restriction in the treatment and prevention of cancer?:
https://www.ncbi.nlm.nih.gov/pmc/articles/PMC3267662/

Last but not least, Dr. Sophia Lunt explains in her TEDx talk, how she intends to cut off cancer cells' survival potential, and describes a new way of halting their growth:

Starving cancer away | Sophia Lunt | TEDxMSU
https://www.youtube.com/watch?v=f6rSuJ2YheQ

Unfortunately, even if there are exceptions, most doctors have no idea of the benefits of fasting on cancer treatments. Even worse, very often, for emotional support, hospital nurses give cookies and candies (pure cancer-feeding foods) as a treat to all the patients. I hope someday, medical schools will teach about health, nutrition, prevention and the human immune system...

Intermittent Fasting (IF) is also a powerful tool. It is an eating pattern that cycles between periods of fasting and eating. IF is based on the theory that fasting has been a practice throughout human evolution and that cycling between periods of "famine" and "feasting" is an ancestrally adapted way of eating for us. Ancient hunter-gatherers didn't have supermarkets, refrigerators or food available every day, year-round. Sometimes they couldn't find anything to eat for days. It is also very probable that our cavemen ancestors often had to "exercise" (hunt, climb trees, run, fight...) on an empty stomach, and the improved cognitive function of fasting undoubtedly helped them to survive and find food. As a result, humans evolved to be able to function without food for extended periods of time... This educated guess made fasted-workouts very popular in the athletic circles over the past ten years.

Some of the most common IF protocols are:

-   The 16:8 protocol: fast for 16h. Eating window is 8h.

-   The Warrior diet: fast for 20h. Eating window is 4h.

-   OMAD (One Meal A Day): fast for 23h. Eating window is 1h.

- OAW (Once A Week) fast: fast for 24h to 48h, once a week.

- 5:2 protocol: eat normally for 5 days and fast for 2 days.

- Alternate Day Fasting: alternate between normal eating days and days of "semi-fast" at 400 to 600 calories.

More and more studies prove the health benefits of IF and that fasting cyclically is more natural than always eating three (or more) meals a day.

I, personally, have been doing IF for more than fifteen years (seriously but not religiously), simply because I feel much better doing my morning workout and martial arts HIIT training on an empty stomach.

When you fast, several things happen in your body at the cellular level; your body adjusts hormone levels to make stored body fat more accessible; your cells also initiate important repair processes and change the expression of genes.

Here are some changes that occur in your body when you fast:

- Human Growth Hormone (HGH): the levels of growth hormone skyrocket, increasing as much as five times. This has benefits for fat loss and muscle gain, to name a few.

Read the study here:

https://www.ncbi.nlm.nih.gov/pmc/articles/PMC329619/

- Insulin: insulin sensitivity improves, and the levels of insulin drop dramatically. Lower insulin levels make stored body fat more accessible for fuel. Insulin is the key to turn on/off fat deposition.

Read the study here:

https://www.ncbi.nlm.nih.gov/pubmed/15640462

- Cellular repair: when fasted, your cells initiate cellular repair processes. This includes autophagy, where cells digest and remove old and dysfunctional proteins that build up inside cells.

Read the study here:

https://www.ncbi.nlm.nih.gov/pmc/articles/PMC3106288/

- Gene expression: there are changes in the function of genes related to longevity and protection against disease and inflammation.

Read the study here:

https://www.ncbi.nlm.nih.gov/pmc/articles/PMC262 2429/

These changes in hormone levels, cell function and gene expression are responsible for the health benefits of IF. Intermittent Fasting is also a powerful tool to lose weight and body fat. It boosts metabolism while helping you naturally eat fewer calories; it keeps your insulin level very low for as long as you are in a fasting period (at least half of the day or more for most people). Spending a big part of your day doing your things with zero fuel from food, you enter a state of ketosis where the body has to use its own body fat to function. If you mix IF with a Keto or low-carb diet, you will turn your body into a fat-burning-furnace.

More studies on both animals and humans have shown that IF can have powerful benefits for weight control and the health of your body and brain. It may even help you live longer.

Here are the general health benefits of Intermittent Fasting:

- Weight loss: as mentioned above, Intermittent Fasting can help you lose weight and belly fat, without having to consciously restrict calories.

- Insulin resistance: Intermittent Fasting can reduce insulin resistance, lowering blood sugar by 3–6% and dropping insulin levels by 20–31%, which could protect against type-2 diabetes

Read the study here:

https://www.sciencedirect.com/science/article/pii/S193152441400200X

- Chronic inflammation: some studies show reductions in inflammation markers, a key driver of many chronic diseases.

Read the study here:

https://www.ncbi.nlm.nih.gov/pubmed/17291990/

- Heart health: both fasting and Intermittent Fasting reduces blood triglycerides, inflammatory markers, blood sugar and insulin resistance — all risk factors for heart disease.

Read the study here:

https://www.ncbi.nlm.nih.gov/pubmed/19793855

- Cancer: animal studies suggest that IF might prevent cancer.

Read the studies here:

https://www.ncbi.nlm.nih.gov/pubmed/22323820

https://www.ncbi.nlm.nih.gov/pubmed/3245934

- Brain health: Intermittent Fasting increases the brain hormone BDNF and may aid the growth of new nerve cells. It may also protect against Alzheimer's disease.

Read the study here:

https://www.ncbi.nlm.nih.gov/pubmed/17306982

- Anti-aging: Intermittent Fasting extends the lifespan of lab rats. Studies showed that fasted rats lived 36–83% longer.

Read the study here:

https://www.karger.com/Article/Abstract/212538

For people recovering from an injury or an operation, a bone broth fast is also very powerful tool.

Studies show that long fasts under medical supervision – from 48h up to 3 weeks – may be of great help in fighting cancer.

French health expert Thierry Casasnovas often talks about one of his friends who completely healed from a stage-4 liver cancer with a 21-day fast as his only treatment. There is a growing body of evidence supporting the role of fasting in both cancer treatment and prevention.

10.   Juicing to help fight cancer

Juicing may seem like just a health fad, but there are real benefits of juicing for people with cancer. According to the American Cancer Society, eating at least 2 cups of vegetables and ½ cup of fruits each day can help to reduce your risk for a variety of cancers because they are rich in antioxidants. Antioxidants have the ability to attack free radicals in the body. Free radicals can damage the DNA in your cells over time, leading to disease. Foods high in antioxidants include carrots, green leafy vegetables, berries, citrus fruits, apples and organic green tea. Because insoluble fibers can be irritating to people with certain cancers, juicing is one of the best ways to get tons of beneficial antioxidant and micro-nutrients without aggravating the inflammation.

A recent review of research published in *Medical News Today* highlighted the health benefits of carrot juice, including the prevention of chronic obstructive pulmonary disease (COPD), breast, stomach and colon cancers, and can prevent side effects from leukemia treatment. Juicing is a great way to get the nutritional benefits of fruits and vegetables without the bulk — 1 cup of carrot juice is nutritionally equal to 5 cups of sliced carrots.

Here is an interesting article on juicing and oncology:

https://www.oncologynutrition.org/erfc/healthy-nutrition-now/foods/should-i-be-juicing

Here are several examples of the juices I did after I was healed (remember that it is critical to use seasonal vegetable and rotate your veggies to avoid oxalates and other phytotoxines poisoning). I personally didn't eat any fruits or root vegetables at all for as long as I was sick but reintroduced some after the tumor was gone.

Those recipes are for one person.

Juice #1:

½ a lettuce
6 carrots
1 red beetroot
1 inch of fresh turmeric (curcumin)

Juice #2:

¼ lbs. of parsley
6 purple carrots
1 beetroot
½ a red apple
1 inch of fresh turmeric (curcumin)

Juice #3:

¼ lbs. of baby spinach
1 handful of blueberries
1 stalk of celery
1 inch of fresh turmeric (curcumin)

Juice #4:

½ a lettuce

6 carrots
1 small piece of fresh ginger
1 inch of fresh turmeric (curcumin)

Juice #5:

¼ lbs. of pak choy
3 stalks of celery
1 red beetroot
1 handful of raspberries
1 inch of fresh turmeric (curcumin)

Juice #6:

8 multi-color carrots
1 lemon
1 inch of fresh turmeric (curcumin)

Juice #7:

¼ lbs. of baby spinach
1 lemon
1 red cabbage
1 inch of fresh turmeric (curcumin)

Juice #8:

¼ lbs. of kale
3 carrots
5 strawberries
1 inch of fresh turmeric (curcumin)

Juice #9 (my favorite):

6 carrots
1 beetroot
½ a lettuce
1 blood orange
1 inch of fresh turmeric (curcumin)

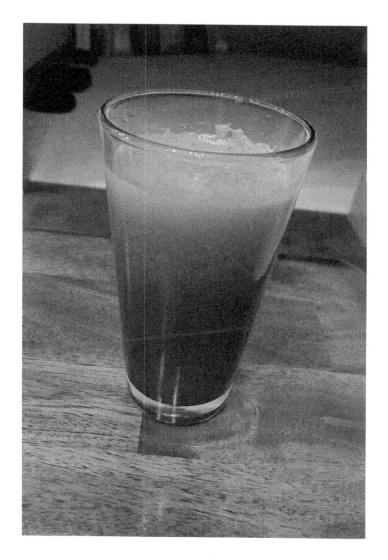

Juice #9

11. Exercise to help fight cancer

Exercise, especially fasted exercise (working-out on an empty stomach), accelerates the elimination/cleansing process of the body, and this is why it was one of the tools I used for my natural healing.

Here is a great article on how exercise can help prevent or fight cancer:

https://www.the-scientist.com/features/regular-exercise-helps-patients-combat-cancer-67317

I will explain my full protocol in detail in chapter 3, but as far as fasted exercise, here what I did: At first, I couldn't even walk so I didn't exercise at all for 2 months. That's when I lost lots of my muscle mass and ended up at 49Kg.

I then started to incorporate 10min. of Tai Chi in every day for a few weeks, until I built enough energy to start doing my HIIT again (High Intensity Interval Training) - based on boxing, rope skipping, push-ups and air squats – 3 to 4 times a week. At that time, I also started teaching martial arts again once in a while, for an hour.

And finally, I was ready to go back to the gym and put some weight back on. I, of course, did all of those trainings on an empty stomach, as I've been doing for the past 15 years, and only broke my fast after my work-outs around 1:30pm.

12. Meditation and breathing to help fight cancer

Meditation has several benefits for people fighting cancer, and many cancer centers now offer it as part of the treatment. Benefits include a reduction in anxiety and depression, reduced stress, greater energy, deeper breathing and a decrease in chronic pain among other symptoms. At the same time, there are pretty much no risks and unlike many complementary treatments used to control the symptoms of cancer, no side effects.

I personally used meditation along with Buddhist mantras and positive visualizations. It really helped me increase my energy, especially what Traditional Chinese Medicine calls "Wei Chi", our defensive energy, and decrease the stress/fear that my way of dealing with cancer could kill me.

Just for those interested, the two Mantras I used, were the *Gayatri* Mantra and the *Om Mani Padme Hum* Mantra.

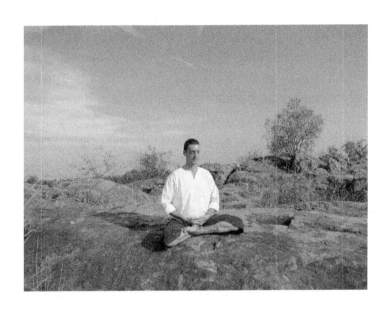

Benefits:

Meditation has many benefits for general health and well-being. It has been found to decrease heart rate, lower blood pressure, ease muscle tension, and improve mood. Emotionally, the practice of meditation has helped many people restore a feeling of calm by centering their thoughts and closing their minds to fears about the future and regrets about the past. But meditation may also have specific benefits for people who are living with cancer. Some of these include:

Depression and Anxiety:

One study found a decrease in symptoms of depression for people with cancer after mindfulness-based cognitive therapy. And unlike some alternative treatments that only have short-term benefits for cancer patients, these effects were still present three months later.

Stress:

Several studies have found meditation to significantly improve the perception of stress in people coping with cancer. This benefit may go beyond the subjective feeling of well-being when stress is reduced, and contribute to a healthier immune system as well. Stress hormones -

chemicals that are released in our bodies when we experience stress - may play a role in how well someone responds to cancer treatment, and even affect survival. One study found that meditation decreased the levels of stress hormones in people with breast and prostate cancer and that the effects were still present a year later. Meditation may also lower the levels of Th1 cytokines, which are inflammatory factors produced by the body that may affect how we respond to cancer and our healing from cancer.

Chronic Pain:

Chronic pain is a common and very frustrating symptom among people with cancer. The cause may be due to cancer itself, due to treatments for cancer, or secondary to other causes. Whatever the cause, it's estimated that roughly 90% of people with lung cancer experience some degree of pain. Meditation appears to help with this pain and may lessen the number of pain medications needed to control pain.

Sleep Problems:

Difficulty with sleep is a common problem for people living with cancer. In several studies, meditation is associated with less insomnia and improved quality of sleep.

Cognitive Functioning:

Difficulty with cognitive functioning is common and may be due to cancer itself or treatments for cancer, such as chemotherapy. Several studies have found meditation to improve cognitive functioning with cancer

Fatigue:

Fatigue is one of the most annoying symptoms of cancer and cancer treatments. Studies suggest that meditation may improve energy levels and lessen fatigue for people living with cancer.

Cancer cells are anaerobic and thrive in a low oxygen environment, and in fact cannot survive in an oxygen-rich environment as evidenced by a 2000 study published in Cancer Research Journal among many other studies.

Here is an interesting study on "Yoga breathing" (Pranayama) and cancer therapies:

https://www.ncbi.nlm.nih.gov/pmc/articles/PMC335 3818/

And another one on meditation, melatonin production and the prevention of breast and prostate cancers:

13. Tai Chi for cancer patients

Tai Chi (aka Tai Chi Chuan or Taiji Quan), is an exercise that originated in ancient China and is a combination of Martial Arts, Traditional Chinese Medicine and Daoist philosophy. The Compendium of Physical Activities assigned a Metabolic Equivalent of task score of 4.0 to Tai Chi, which is classified as moderate intensity activity. Yet in older adults and adults with health conditions, Tai Chi is frequently carried out in a gentle and non-strenuous form making it potentially suitable for cancer patients. Moreover, compared with other forms of Qigong, Tai Chi is better suited for cancer survivors, owing to the simplicity and slowness of the movements involved with the exercise.

Chinese Tai Chi has been shown to reduce inflammation that is linked with many chronic diseases, including heart disease and cancer. Several studies show that Tai Chi improves balance which may also help to reduce the risk of falls. Clinical trials suggest that Tai Chi can help reduce fatigue in breast cancer patients.

Here is a study on the potential yield of Tai Chi in cancer survivorship:

https://www.ncbi.nlm.nih.gov/pmc/articles/PMC5242198/

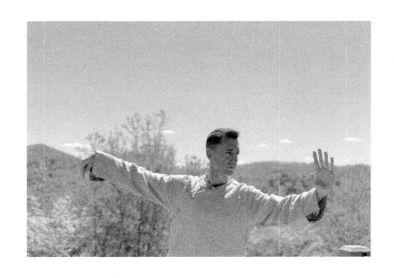

14. Rebounding on a mini-trampoline to help fight cancer

- Rebounding stimulates lymph circulation – a very good thing for healing cancer

Lymph starts its life as plasma in arterial blood. When the blood filters through tissue to deliver nutrients to cells and remove waste products, not all of it returns to the circulatory system. The 10% or so that is left behind becomes lymph and moves through the lymphatic system up towards the neck before it's dumped back into the bloodstream at the subclavian veins. Along the way it gets filtered by the lymph nodes and any nasties are attacked by white blood cells. According to the Ehrlich Lymph Organization, *"Lymph nodes also trap and destroy cancer cells to slow the spread of cancer until they are overwhelmed by it."*

Having a highly functioning lymphatic system is essential for your overall health and ability to fight cancer. The lymphatic system is comprised of several organs including the spleen, tonsils and lymph nodes, which are interconnected by a web of fine lymphatic vessels. The lymphatic system receives toxins and metabolic waste which are transported by the lymphatic fluid to the lymph nodes, to be discharged to the kidneys and liver for elimination. So, without the lymphatic system, the body cannot effectively remove toxins.

The body has three times as much lymph as it does blood. But whereas the circulatory system has the heart to pump blood through the body, the lymphatic system depends purely on the movement of muscles and joints to move that fluid around. The rebounding action of a mini-trampoline is especially effective at moving lymph towards the nodes on its way to being filtered and detoxified. The flow of lymph is controlled by one-way valves that prevent backflow. In the absence of a pump, the motion of the rebounder helps coordinate the opening and closing of those valves so things move along nicely.

- Rebounding boosts the immune system – another very good thing for healing cancer

Circulating lymph makes it easier for the immune system to eliminate all the wastes and toxins. Not only does healthy lymph movement push waste towards lymph nodes for processing, jumping on a mini-trampoline activates human lymphocytes (specialized white blood cells which research suggests can kill tumor cells). In fact, these are the same white blood cells that are leveraged by some immunotherapy protocols. After only two minutes of jumping on a trampoline the number of white blood cells triples and remains elevated for up to an hour.

- Rebounding increases oxygen intake – again, a very good thing for healing cancer

As we saw before, cancer cells are anaerobic and thrive in a low oxygen environment and in fact cannot survive in an oxygen-rich environment as evidenced by a 2000 study published in Cancer Research Journal among many other studies. One important tool as we "tend the soil" of our bodies to create a cancer-hostile environment by saturating our tissues with oxygen.

15. Extreme cold exposure / cryotherapy

Cryotherapy uses extreme cold to strengthen the immune system and, in some cases, destroy cancer cells. In those cases, during cryotherapy treatment, the doctor freezes the cancer cells to kill them. Cold strengthening can be used different ways and via three possible vectors: in a cryotherapy chamber, in water or via the air:

1. In a chamber where the temperature drops to −110°C through the injection of nitrogen air (1 to 3 minutes)

2. Extreme cold in water at -5°C for a short time (30 seconds to 2 minutes)

3. Moderate cold by air for longer periods (20 to 30 minutes outside at 0°C

Read a few studies on the subject:

Cancer Cryotherapy: Evolution and Biology

https://www.ncbi.nlm.nih.gov/pmc/articles/PMC147 2868/

Exposure to extreme cold can also help cancer patients by reducing inflammation, as shown in this study

https://www.ncbi.nlm.nih.gov/pmc/articles/PMC541 1446/

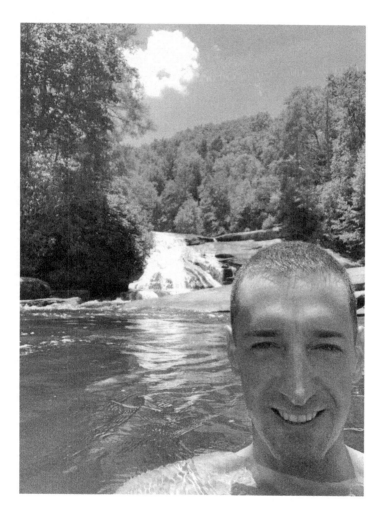

Cold exposure to boost the immune system - in the mountains' waterfalls - water at 3°C (37°F)

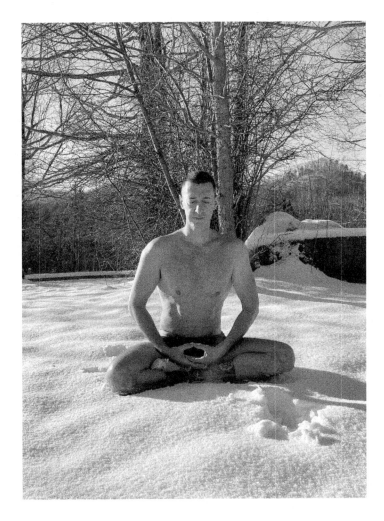

15 minutes meditation in the snow

16.   Psychotherapy and cancer

Since the very beginning I wanted to "attack" the cancer from every possible angles. A real holistic approach, physical, physiological, mental, emotional, energetical and spiritual. That is why I used fasting, juicing, Ketogenic dieting, but also fasted exercise, HIIT, Tai Chi, meditation, rebounding, breathing, ice-cold bathes, stretching and... psychotherapy.

I never really thought or felt that I needed to do a therapy, but in my research, it was one of the tools often mentioned by people who chose the natural approach. So, I jumped into it. I called my friend Doctor Charles Gibert (a French MD, acupuncturist, homeopath and psychotherapist), to dig deeper into my personal history, eventual traumas and family emotional history. To my complete surprise, I learned a lot about myself, but also about my dad, my mon, my grand-parents and their lives in Nazi "working camps" during World War II, and much more...

It is hard to say if this had a direct link with my healing (even though I do think so), but it sure was interesting and made me a better person.

17.   Faith and the Law of Attraction

Even though faith was a big part of my journey (spiritual faith but also faith in nature, in the immune system, in my body's ability to heal...), it is not my goal to talk about religion here (I wrote other books for that), but I will talk a little bit about the spiritual Law of Attraction as it is one of the main tools that I used to heal myself.

The Law of Attraction is the belief that positive or negative thoughts bring positive or negative experiences into a person's life. The belief is based on the ideas that people and their thoughts are made from "pure energy", and that a process of like-energy attracting like-energy exists through which a person can improve their health, wealth, relationships, and personal life. The Law of Attraction is most obvious in Buddhism, and there many of the Buddha's quotes that refers to it, such as:

"What you think, you become. What you feel, you attract. What you imagine, you can create".

But there are traces of the law of attraction in every religion, and here is another example from the Jewish Talmud:

"Pay *attention to your thoughts, they will become your words.*

"*Pay attention to your words, they will become acts.*

"*Pay attention to your acts, they will become habits.*

"*Pay attention to your habits, they will become your character.*

"*Pay attention to your character, because it is your destiny.*"

In the Bible, in Mark 11:24, it is said: *"Therefore I tell you, whatever you ask in prayer, believe that you have received it already and it will be yours."*

In my personal battle against cancer, in my daily meditation, I used the prayer: *"I am thankful for my full and final healing. I am healed and healthy."*

18. Love

It might sound obvious, but to have the full support of your loved one is critical in the healing process. I am so lucky that my wife, my family and all my close friends had total faith in me and in my way of thinking. Not once did one of them told me I was crazy, or even pushed me to go for a "regular" allopathic treatment.

My wife Lila especially was absolutely phenomenal during those hard times. She took over all my martial arts classes, had to take a side job because our businesses were hurt by covid-19, she took care of me, supported me, took care of the house, of the dog, and never ever complained. She cried only one time during those four months, and that was the day I called her from France to tell her I had cancer. What a Warrior she is.

My mother was also incredible and supported each of my decision. She was there for me like only a mother can be, and also played a big part in my healing.

Finally, my dog Kali knew there was something wrong. He also knew exactly where the tumor was, and was a fantastic emotional support. Dogs are incredible and as I am writing those lines, Kali is being trained by a professional to be a Service Dog for cancer detection and emotional support.

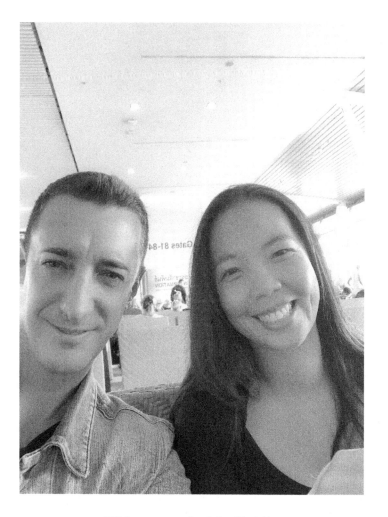

With my wonderful wife Lila

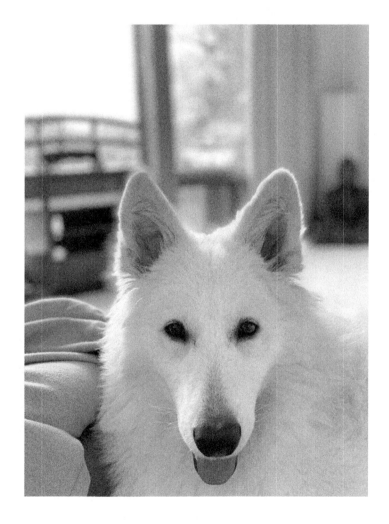

Our White Swiss Shepherd, Kali

Part 3
My protocol

1.   My daily protocol:

Again, I am not a doctor and I am not trying to convince anyone to follow this. This is only the result of my research and it worked for me... without any side effects.

6am: Intermittent Fasting until 2pm (dry fast)
Cold exposure #1 -> 20min. outside in my underwear at 0°C (32°F)

7am: Meditation / deep breathing / Tai Chi

9am: HIIT 3 to 4 times a week / 3min. of mini-trampoline everyday

10am:
- → Cold exposure #2 -> Ice-cold bath to boost the immune system and reduce inflammation. I do mine in mountain waterfalls 3 times a week and in the shower (not as cold) the rest of the time)
- → Once a week -> Psychotherapy
- → Once every two weeks -> Full body massage
- → Once a month -> Chiropractic session

12pm: Workout (weight lifting or CrossFit) 4 times a week (45min. sessions).

2pm: Starting in November (month 3), I added vegetable juices to my Red-Meat-Only diet. I then

break my fast with a fresh vegetable juice (made with organic, seasonal, fresh and local vegetables) and broccoli sprouts
+ Vit D3 -> 20,000 iu with 200 mcg of vit. K2
+ Vit C -> 4 gr
+ Turmeric -> 1 tsp
+ Zinc -> 30 mg
+ Omega 3 (fish oil) : 1000 mg + DHA 500

3pm: Wheatgrass juice mixed with Matcha tea

4pm: Ketogenic meal: usually organic, 100% grass-fed ribeye steak + garlic + olive oil
+ Vit D3 -> 10,000 iu with 100 mcg of vit. K2
+ Vit C -> 2 gr
+ Turmeric -> 1 tsp
+ Digestive enzymes
+ Bromelain : 1000 mg
+ Alpha Lipoic Acid : 1200 mg
+ Garcinia Cambogia : 3200 mg

4:30pm: Macha green tea (just after red meat to minimize the absorption of glutamine)
+ 30 mg of melatonin

Start Intermittent Fasting until 2pm the next day

9:30pm: Bed time

2. My anti-cancer diet over a week

Sunday: 36 hours of dry fasting (from Saturday after dinner to Monday morning 10am)

Monday to Friday: Strict zero carb Keto diet (100% grass-fed and grass-finished beef with butter, salt and water at first, and with adding veggie juices after a few months) when I was sick, and after February 2021, a modified ketogenic diet with juices slightly higher in carbs (carrots, beetroots, blueberries, etc.)

Saturday: After February, one "cheat meal" once month - non-ketogenic with varied and seasonal fruits, and possibly carbs such as potatoes or rice (previously soaked for 12 hours)

Done! 4 months to beat the cancer, without long chemotherapy (3 sessions only), without radiation and without the surgery described as essential by oncologists if I wanted to live.

I would like to make it clear that I am aware that I was in the perfect environment to be able to do what I did, and that it does not mean that I am pushing others to do like me. I live in the Blue Ridge Mountains of South Carolina, where there is low pollution, little crime, no noise, mountains and trees all around my house, icy waterfalls minutes from the home...

I also had the support of my family including my fantastic wife, and most importantly, I didn't have to go to work for four months (I have developed a martial arts school franchise, with amazing teams that have allowed me to focus solely and totally on my healing).

Part 4
Ketogenic recipes

For those who haven't read my book on the Ketogenic diet *"Eat fat to lose fat - the French paradox"*, here are some of the keto recipes I shared in it and that I use as an anti-cancer keto diet. There are a lot more on the Keto book, which you can find here:

https://www.amazon.com/Eat-Fat-Lose-French-Paradox/dp/1081493925/ref=sr_1_7?dchild=1&keywords=fred+evrard&qid=1609603692&sr=8-7

If for any reason you cannot buy organic, be aware of the EWG's Dirty Dozen, the twelve worst pesticide-heavy foods to eat:

1. *Strawberries*
2. *Spinach*
3. *Kale*
4. *Nectarines*
5. *Apples*
6. *Grapes*
7. *Peaches*
8. *Cherries*
9. *Pears*
10. *Tomatoes*
11. *Celery*
12. *Potatoes*

The following recipes are for four persons, but of course, if it seems too much or too little for you and your family, adapt the portions to your appetite. Stop eating when you are full, but make sure you have enough daily calories, fats and proteins. A lot of people, when starting a Ketogenic diet do not eat enough because the fat fills them up more than the carbs.

I.   French influence

- **Slow cooked pork or lamb shoulder "à la cuillère"**

Ingredients:
1 bone-in shoulder of pork or lamb
2 tbsp. of organic cold-pressed olive oil
3 tbsp. of organic 100% grass-fed butter
6 cups of bone broth
Pink Himalayan salt
Pepper
Garlic powder
Onion powder

Preparation and cooking:
Remove meat from fridge 1h. before cooking.

20min. before cooking brush with olive oil then season with salt, pepper, garlic and onion powder on both sides.

In a sauté pan, brown the meat in butter or ghee on all sides at high temperature.

Then lower the temperature to the minimum, cover the meat with bone broth, cover and cook for 3h. (lamb) or 4h. (pork). Half way through, flip the meat to the other side. Baste the meat with its bone broth every 30min. to prevent it from drying out.

Note about butter: High quality butter is golden-yellow in color. If it's white or light color, it's probably low quality, processed and grain-fed.

- **"Poulet à la crème", creamy chicken with mushrooms**

Ingredients:
8 boneless chicken thighs with skin
1 tbsp. of organic 100% grass-fed ghee
1 cup of organic grass fed heavy cream
Pink Himalayan salt
Pepper
Garlic powder
Onion powder
3 cups of fresh organic mushrooms, minced

Preparation and cooking:
Remove meat from fridge 30min. before cooking.

20min. before cooking, brush with olive oil, then season with salt, pepper, garlic and onion powder on both sides.

In a sauté pan, brown the meat in butter or ghee on all sides at high temperature.

Then lower the temperature to the minimum, cover the meat with the heavy cream, add the minced mushrooms, cover and cook for 20min.

- "Cote de bœuf 2 cuissons" Bone-in Ribeye cooked twice

<u>Ingredients</u>:
1 extra thick grass-fed bone-in Ribeye (2.5 inches thick or more)
2 tbsp. of organic 100% grass-fed butter or ghee
2 tbsp. of organic cold-pressed olive oil
Pink Himalayan salt
Pepper
Garlic powder
Onion powder
Herbs of your choice (thyme, oregano...)

<u>Preparation and cooking</u>:
Remove meat from fridge 1h. before cooking.

Brush with olive oil, then season with salt, pepper, garlic and onion powder on both sides.

In a sauté pan, brown the meat in butter or ghee on all sides at high temperature.

Pre-heat your oven to 400°F (200°C).

Put the meat in an oven safe baking dish (or even better, a cast-iron pan if you have one). Cook for about 6min. per pound (see chart below).

VERY IMPORTANT: Red meat needs to "rest" for about 8min. before serving. It's going to be much juicer and more tender. Add butter and "fleur de sel de Guérande" ET VOILA!

SIRLOIN STRIP STEAKS, RIBEYE STEAKS & PORTERHOUSE STEAKS

Thickness	Rare 110° To 120° F	Medium Rare 120° To 130° F	Medium 130° To 140° F
1"	4 minutes EACH SIDE	5 minutes EACH SIDE	6 minutes EACH SIDE
1.25"	4.5 minutes EACH SIDE	5.5 minutes EACH SIDE	6.5 minutes EACH SIDE
1.5"	5 minutes EACH SIDE	6 minutes EACH SIDE	7 minutes EACH SIDE
1.75"	5.5 minutes EACH SIDE	6.5 minutes EACH SIDE	7.5 minutes EACH SIDE
2"	6 minutes EACH SIDE	7 minutes EACH SIDE	8 minutes EACH SIDE

- Crustless French quiche

Ingredients:
5 organic eggs
250 ml. of organic heavy cream
1/2 lbs. of sugar-free bacon
1 cup of organic grass-fed grated Swiss cheese (you could use cheddar but remember that it's one of the most processed cheese out there)
Pink Himalayan salt
Pepper

Preparation and cooking:
Cut and pre-cook the bacon in a pan and set aside.

Mix the eggs with the cream in a food processor.

Mix all ingredients together (reserving ¼ cup of cheese) and put everything in a deep-dish pie pan, cover with the reserved cheese.

Cook at 300°F (150°C) for 30-40min. until golden-brown.

Let the quiche rest for 20min. Enjoy!

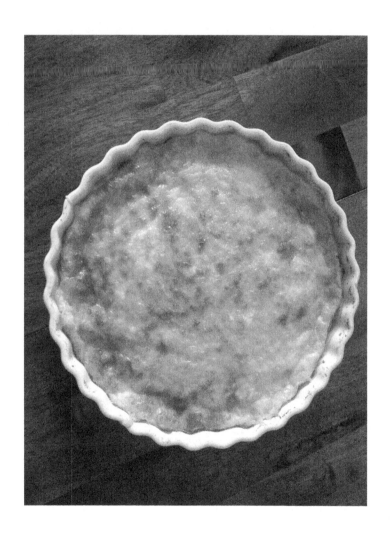

II.   Asian influence

- **Thai lemongrass chicken thighs with cauliflower rice**

Ingredients:
Organic free-range boneless chicken thighs with skin
3 tbsp. of organic coconut oil
1 clove of organic garlic
Sugar-free Thai red curry paste
2 chopped stalks of lemongrass
Fresh Cilantro
3 kaffir lime leaves
Pink Himalayan salt

Preparation and cooking:
Marinate the chicken with the red curry paste, the chopped lemongrass, chopped Cilantro and the chopped kaffir lime leaves in the fridge overnight.

Get the marinated chicken out of the fridge 20min. before cooking it.

In a sauté pan, brown the thighs in coconut oil on skin side at high temperature until skin is crispy.

Then lower the temperature, flip the thighs, add the garlic and cook the other side for another 2-3min.

- "Fong Kai" Hakka-style red chicken

Ingredients:
Organic free-range boneless chicken thighs with skin
3 tbsp. of organic coconut oil
1 clove of organic garlic
Sugar-free red chili pepper sauce
¼ cup of gluten-free organic Tamari or soy sauce
Pink Himalayan salt
1 tsp. of Chinese 5-spice powder
½ gallon of homemade bone broth

Preparation and cooking:
Remove meat from fridge 30min. before cooking.

In a large stockpot, brown the thighs in coconut oil on both sides at high temperature until skin is crispy.

Lower the temperature, add the garlic, chili sauce, salt, Chinese 5-spice and soy sauce, cover everything with bone broth.

Cover the pan and cook for another 1h.

Serve the red chicken in a bowl with the cooking liquid, and sides of cauliflower rice and sautéed Pak Choy.

- **Thai coconut green curry with duck**

Ingredients:
4 free-range duck breasts with skin
1 tbsp. of organic coconut oil
Sugar-free Thai green curry paste
2 cups of organic coconut cream
2 chopped kaffir lime leaves
Pink Himalayan salt
16 baby Thai eggplants (cut in half)

Preparation and cooking:
Get the duck out of the fridge 30min. before cooking it.

In a sauté pan, brown the thighs in coconut oil on both sides at high temperature, until skin is crispy.

Transfer duck to a large saucepan and add remaining ingredients. Cook over low heat for 20min. until eggplants are fully cooked (they should be soft)

- Vietnamese low-carb Pho soup

Ingredients:
Homemade bone broth
4 8-oz. grass-fed beef filet
1 lbs. of grass-fed beef brisket
4 packages of organic shirataki "miracle noodles"
1 clove of organic garlic, minced
2 onions, sliced
4 spring onion butts
3 star anise
2 cloves
1/3 cup of organic gluten-free soy sauce
Pink Himalayan salt
Fresh cilantro
Fresh basil
2 handfuls of soybean sprouts

Preparation and cooking:
Cut the filet into thin slices and marinate with the garlic, 1 onion, soy sauce and salt in the fridge for at least 1h.

Remove the marinated beef from the fridge 1h. before putting it in the soup.

Rinse the shirataki noodle very carefully, cook them in salted boiling water and dry them in a pan as indicated in the directions. Set aside.

Cook the brisket in the bone broth together with star anise, cloves and spring onion butts. When brisket is cooked, remove the ingredients.

Put the noodles in 4 separate large bowls. Put raw beef and cooked brisket on top and pour in the very hot broth. Add remaining onion, basil, cilantro and soybean sprouts. Enjoy!

III.   International influence

-   **Organic bunless cheeseburger**

<u>Ingredients</u>:
3lbs. of organic grass fed ground beef (preferably 75% lean 25% fat)
1 tbsp. of organic ghee
Pink Himalayan salt
Pepper
Garlic powder
Onion powder
8 slices of organic raw-milk Swiss cheese
8 large lettuce wraps
1 organic tomato
Organic guacamole (homemade if possible)

<u>Preparation and cooking</u>:
Prepare your patties with ground beef, salt, onion and garlic powder (I usually count 0.75lbs. per person but not everyone eats as much as I do...)

Grill the burger on an outdoor grill - or in a frying pan with ghee - on one side. Flip them and immediately add the cheese so it has time to melt.

Prepare your lettuce wraps with the guacamole and slices of tomatoes. Put the patties with melted cheese on top. Enjoy!

- **Grilled Ribeye, mashed "ketatoes" and asparagus**

Ingredients:
4 thick grass-fed Ribeyes (2 inches thick)
2 tbsp. of organic cold-pressed olive oil
Pink Himalayan salt
Guérande fleur de sel
Pepper
Garlic powder
Onion powder
Asparagus

For the mashed "ketatoes":
2 heads of organic cauliflower, cut into florets
2 tbsp. of 100% grass-fed butter
1 cup of 100% grass-fed heavy cream
½ cup of organic cream cheese
Enough bone broth to cook the cauliflower
2 garlic cloves, minced
Pink Himalayan salt
Pepper

Preparation and cooking:
Remove meat from the fridge 1h. before cooking.

20min. before cooking, brush the ribeyes and the asparagus with olive oil and season with salt, pepper, garlic and onion powder.

Pre-heat your BBQ grill to 400°F (200°C).

Cook the Ribeyes to your liking (using the chart below).

3min. before meat is done put the asparagus on the grill.

Let the meat rest for 8min. before serving.

For the garlic mashed "ketatoes":

Put the cauliflower, salt and broth in a large pot. Cover and cook until the cauliflower is tender.

Drain the liquid, and squeeze excess from the cauliflower by placing it between 2 paper towels. Get as much as liquid out as possible for a better "mashed potato" effect.

In a food processor, combine the cooked cauliflower with all the cream, butter, cream cheese, garlic, salt and pepper. Purée until smooth.

Better prepare the mashed "ketatoes" before cooking the meat and reheat before eating.

SIRLOIN STRIP STEAKS, RIBEYE STEAKS & PORTERHOUSE STEAKS

Thickness	Rare 110° To 120° F	Medium Rare 120° To 130° F	Medium 130° To 140° F
1"	4 minutes EACH SIDE	5 minutes EACH SIDE	6 minutes EACH SIDE
1.25"	4.5 minutes EACH SIDE	5.5 minutes EACH SIDE	6.5 minutes EACH SIDE
1.5"	5 minutes EACH SIDE	6 minutes EACH SIDE	7 minutes EACH SIDE
1.75"	5.5 minutes EACH SIDE	6.5 minutes EACH SIDE	7.5 minutes EACH SIDE
2"	6 minutes EACH SIDE	7 minutes EACH SIDE	8 minutes EACH SIDE

VERY IMPORTANT: Red meat needs to "rest" 6-8min. before serving. It's going to be much juicer and more tender. Add a butter and "fleur de sel" and enjoy!

- **Unilateral salmon**

Ingredients:
4 thick wild caught salmon fillets with skin
2 tbsp. of organic cold-pressed olive or avocado oil
Pink Himalayan salt
Pepper
1 lemon

Preparation and cooking:
Remove salmon from the fridge 15min. before cooking. Season with salt and pepper.

In a sauté pan on medium heat, cook the salmon in oil on skin side only. DO NOT FLIP IT. When you can see from the sides that the fillet is cooked halfway through, the salmon is ready.

Serve on 4 plates. Squeeze fresh lemon juice on top.

Enjoy your meal.

- **Keto cobb salad**

Ingredients:
8 cups of organic lettuce or mixed green salad
4 organic eggs
2 cups of cherry tomatoes
1/2 lbs. of sugar-free bacon
1 cup of organic Roquefort (French sheep-milk blue cheese)
4 organic avocados
Pink Himalayan salt
Pepper
Organic cold-pressed olive oil
Organic apple cider vinegar

Preparation and cooking:
Soft boil the eggs and let them cool down.

Cut and pre-cook the bacon in a pan.

Cut/slice all ingredients.

Put everything in a large bowl, cover with a little extra cheese.

Prepare your vinaigrette with the oil, vinegar, salt and pepper – Ratio is 2tbsp. of oil for 1tbsp. of vinegar.

- African chicken stew with coconut cauliflower rice

Ingredients:
4 organic free-range chicken leg quarters with skin
4 ripe organic tomatoes
½ cup + 1 tbsp. of organic coconut cream
3 tbsp. of organic coconut oil
1 tsp. of curry powder
1 tsp. of paprika
1 tsp. of onion powder
1 large onion
1 clove of garlic, minced
1 tbsp. of organic peanut butter
1 handful of scallions, chopped
Pink Himalayan salt
Pepper
Thyme
2 cups of homemade bone broth
½ cup of shredded coconut (dry)
Cauliflower rice

Preparation and cooking:
Remove chicken from the fridge 20min. before cooking. With a knife, separate thighs and drumsticks

In a large stockpot, brown the thighs in coconut oil (2 tbsp.) on both sides at high temperature until skin is crispy. Set aside.

Using the same pot (without washing it) put the tomatoes, onion, minced garlic, curry powder, paprika and thyme and cook them for 10min.

Add the bone broth, the peanut butter and ½ cup coconut cream. Mix everything well and add the chicken.

Cover and cook everything at low temperature for 30min.

For the coconut cauliflower rice:
Sauté the rice in coconut oil (1 tbsp.) with shredded coconut and 1 tbsp. of coconut cream. Salt to your liking.

Put the rice and stew in one or two separate bowls (up to you), add the scallions on top of the chicken stew. Enjoy!

IV.   Desserts

-    **Keto Pancakes**

<u>Ingredients</u>:
6 oz. of organic cream cheese, softened
1.5 cups of almond flour
1 cup of coconut flour
6 organic eggs
1 tsp. of organic powdered swerve
1/4 tsp. of Himalayan pink salt
4 tbsp. of organic raw coconut oil
Organic 100% grass-fed butter

<u>Preparation and baking</u>:
Blend all ingredients in a food processor or blender.

In a 6-inch frying pan, heat coconut oil and cook pancakes on both sides until golden brown

Put them in a plate and add the butter between each pancake. Enjoy!

- Keto chocolate chip cookies

Ingredients:
2 cups almond flour
½ tsp. baking powder
½ tsp. baking soda
½ tsp. pink Himalayan salt
½ cup butter
¼ cup swerve
2 tbsp. heavy cream
1 organic egg
1 tsp. of vanilla powder
1 cup of sugar-free chocolate chips (I use Lily's)

Preparation and baking:
In a bowl, whisk together almond flour, baking powder and baking soda, and salt. Set aside.

Mix together butter softened and the swerve using a food processor.

Beat in the egg. Mix in heavy cream and vanilla and add to the butter/swerve in the food processor. Slowly add the dry ingredients.

Once combined, mix in the chocolate chips.

Refrigerate the dough for 30min.

Scoop into 1-inch balls and place them on a cooking sheet. Press them with your palm to give them a cookie shape.

Bake at 350°F (180°C) for 15 min. (bake until edges are brown).

Let them cool down on the baking tray for 5min. before transferring to a plate.

- Crustless French lemon meringue pie

Ingredients:
6 organic eggs (yolks for the custard and whites for the meringue)
Juice of 4 organic lemons
1 cup of grass-fed butter
½ cup granulated swerve
½ cup powdered swerve

Preparation and baking:
Mix egg yolks, granulated swerve, butter and lemon juice in a double boiler over low heat. Stir until it thickens. Set aside to cool down.

In a large bowl, beat the egg whites with the powdered swerve to firm peaks.

Preheat oven to 370°F (190°C).

Pour warm filling into small individual ramequins, dollop with meringue and spread right to the edges.

Bake 15min. until meringue peaks are golden and firm. Leave another 10min. in the oven turned off.

Then refrigerate for at least 4 hours.

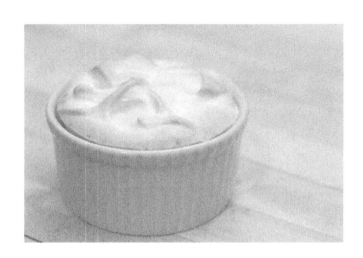

Conclusion

Some people, mostly on social medias, didn't believe me when I said that I was betting on my immune system more than on a full allopathic toxic treatment to heal from cancer. I don't think they will be open minded enough to read this book, but if they do, they will learn and understand that it is not only possible, but that many people did it before me and that many doctors and researchers support natural non-toxic treatments.

I put my faith into what I have been teaching my martial arts students for years, and it worked. As difficult and frightening as this experience was, I am happy to have won this fight and to be a living proof that what I preach works.

I will conclude this testimonial with my "New Year's Eve thought of the day" which I post on my Facebook page on December 31st, 2020:

"This is it. Last day of 2020, finally.

"It's been a challenging year for most of us, and we all lost a lot.

"We've lost people we love, we lost our businesses, we lost time and money, we lost our health, we lost our

ability to travel, and little by little, we're losing our freedom.

"FREEDOM... 2021 is around the corner, and there are still people stupid enough to believe that there is only one way... their way.

"Yes, in the 21st century, there are still people believing that if you're not a Christian, you're going to hell. There are also people who kill in the name of Allah, cutting people's throats simply because they are not Muslims. (I have absolutely nothing against Christians or Muslims. I just have a problem with extremists and terrorists.) There are people who think their martial arts is the best and there is nothing for them in other systems. There are people who believe that there is no healing outside of modern allopathic medicine. They don't believe in nature, they don't believe the immune system can do the job of protecting us, and they want to push their billion-dollar industry medical drugs and vaccines on us. There is more than one way. Nature can heal us, but sometimes we need the surgery; sometimes we don't have time and we need the drugs. And that's fine. There's always a time when we need another path. There's always a time when we need to think differently. There is more than one way and we have to accept it. There are also people who believe that their political party is the only way, whatever the time, whatever the crises. And they are of course

people who will do anything for us to keep thinking that way. The unique thought; the unique way; so they can keep making billions of dollars on our back while we don't ask questions.

"2021 will be interesting. Will it be the year we lose more freedom, more of our ability to think by yourself, or will it be the year of change? Change for the better; change for the environment; change for our health, change for our freedom, change for our happiness.... Time will tell.

"We're all different, and we should embrace it. THERE IS MORE THAN ONE PATH! Happy New Year everyone."

It is now December 2021 as I rewrite and proofread this book for the second edition. We have to admit that we are losing more and more our rights as citizens and our freedom. Freedom of expression - especially concerning the covid-19 crisis and the quasi-forced vaccination that follows - is in real danger. Big Pharma controls (and corrupts) research, politics and all too often the medias.

In 2009, Pfizer was fined $2.3 billion for charlatanism, manipulation of the research and corruption. And they are the ones who decide that their vaccines (they are pushing the 4th dose at the moment) is the only solution to covid-19... What a joke!

(Source: violation tracker)

We failed to embrace the change, and fear once again controls and manipulates the people. Let pray and see what happens in 2022 ...

Appendix: Dogs and cancer

Dogs currently have the highest rate of cancer of any animals on the planet. In the US, one dog out of two is overweight and current canine cancer rates are 1:1.65. Despite advancements in veterinary health care, life expectancy for our pets is declining and dogs nowadays die seven years younger than twenty years ago, and diet is one of the leading causes. Just like for us humans, the causes are mostly environmental but the "food" they eat is probably number one.

Dogs are carnivores, and just as cows are supposed to eat grass and not corn, dogs are supposed to eat meat and not cereals. Kibbles are junk food, period! Even the "top of the line". Imagine a human living exclusively on industrial burgers his entire life... How healthy would he be? Well, kibbles are just that... but ten times worst. They are highly processed, dehydrated, and made of mostly grains (which are very bad for dogs), food preservatives, and the little proteins they contain are of super low quality. There is a reason why they write "for animals only; not for human consumption" on kibble boxes. They wouldn't do that if it was clean and healthy food.

Feeding your pets in general and dogs in particular a BARF diet (Biologically-Adapted Raw Food) is the best thing you can do for your best friend. It's a bit more expensive than kibbles, but you will save tons of money on vet bills and "pets insurance".

Of course, just like humans, food is not their only cause of cancer. Inactivity is also a big one. Your dog should be outside walking, running and playing at the VERY LEAST 2 hours a day. Going for a walk 15min. in the morning and 15min. in the evening just to "go to the bathroom" is not enough. It will drive him crazy, change his behavior and eventually kill him.

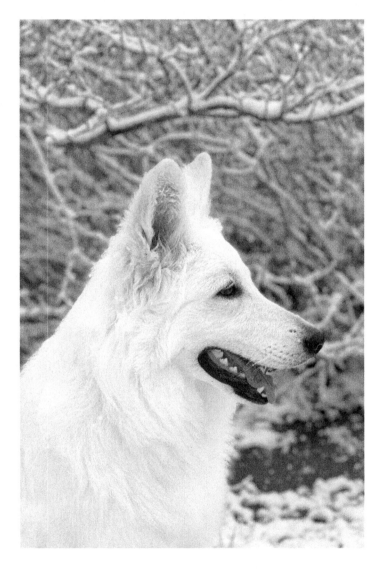

My boy Kali only eats organic, raw meat, organ-meat and bones. He's super healthy and never goes to the vet.

Bibliography

- Cancer as a metabolic disease, *Dr. Thomas N. Seyfried*

- Keto for Cancer: Ketogenic Metabolic Therapy as a Targeted Nutritional Strategy, *Miriam Kalamian, EdM, MS, CNS*

-The metabolic approach to cancer, *Dr. Nasha Winters*

- Des Fiu et des Hommes, *Dr. Charles Gibert*

- Eat fat to lose fat, *Fred Evrard*

- Fat for Fuel: A Revolutionary Diet to Combat Cancer, *Dr. Joseph Mercola*

- Guérir enfin du cancer: Oser dire quand et comment, *Pr. Henry Joyeux*

- Keto answers, *Anthony Gustin, MD and Chris Irvin*

- Lies my doctor told me, *Dr. Ken Berry*

- The Art and Science of Low Carbohydrate Living, *Dr. Stephen Phinney and Dr. Jeff Volek*

- The Wheat Belly, *Dr. William Davis*

- Vous êtes fous d'avaler ça, *Christophe Brusset*

Resources for further research

Doctor Thomas N. Seyfried - Cancer as a Metabolic Disease:
https://www.amazon.com/Cancer-Metabolic-Disease-Management-Prevention/dp/0470584920/ref=sr_1_2?dchild=1&keywords=Thomas+N.+Seyfried+Cancer+as+a+Metabolic+Disease&qid=1609520808&sr=8-2

Doctor Ken D. Berry, MD:
https://www.youtube.com/channel/UCIma2WOQs1Mz2AuOt6wRSUw

Doctor Eric Berg:
https://www.youtube.com/c/DrEricBergDC

Doctor Dominic D'Agostino:
https://www.ketonutrition.org

Thierry Casasnovas / Regenere:
https://www.youtube.com/channel/UCbwkSuFmwbalyCOrwXAtSXA

The Magic Pill documentary (trailer – full documentary on Netflix):
https://www.youtube.com/watch?v=61GitUC_678

About the author – By Lila Evrard

Fred Evrard is a French martial arts instructor, entrepreneur and international speaker on topics such as martial arts, nutrition, natural health, philosophy, comparative religion studies or freemasonry. Fred is the founder of the internationally recognized martial arts system Kali Majapahit and co-founder of counter-terrorism program R.E.D. (Recognize & Escape Danger).

Fred's life is as rich as it is unusual. He started martial arts at the age of six and began to travel the world early on. At seventeen, he was in China studying martial arts and being introduced to Chan Buddhism, Taoism and Meditation. At age twenty-eight while living in Tahiti, he discovered Traditional Chinese medicine with Dr. Charles Gibert, as well as Freemasonry and the European esoteric authors of the 18th and 19th centuries. In 2003, Fred and his wife Lila started a four-year trip around the world during which they had the opportunity to meet amazing people and mentors in Hawaii, Japan, Hong Kong, China, Tibet, Vietnam, Thailand, France, Germany, Sweden, the USA, Lebanon, Canada, the Philippines, Singapore and India. They then lived in Singapore for 10 years and moved to the US in 2016. To this day, Fred and Lila continue to travel the world for both, learning and teaching.

After almost forty years of martial arts practice and twenty-five years studying different traditional healing systems such as Chinese medicine, acupuncture, osteopathy, nutrition and meditation, Fred continues his research and always keeps an open mind to improve his programs.

Fred is also a counter-terrorism consultant for the French Ministry of Defense and a close-quarter-combat trainer for several law enforcement agencies around the world including the French Special Forces.

Books from the same author

The Warrior Monk – From Martial Arts to Martial Hearts

https://www.amazon.fr/Warrior-Monk-Martial-Arts-Hearts/dp/1521769893/ref=sr_1_17?_mk_fr_FR=ÅMÅŽÕÑ&dc hild=1&keywords=Fred+Evrard&qid=1612023803&sr=8-17

Quite smoking, it's easy!

https://www.amazon.fr/Quit-Smoking-its-Easy-effective/dp/1795428244/ref=sr_1_13?_mk_fr_FR=ÅMÅŽÕÑ& dchild=1&keywords=Fred+Evrard&qid=1612023803&sr=8-13

Eat fat to lose fat – The French paradox

https://www.amazon.fr/Eat-Fat-Lose-French-Paradox/dp/1081493925/ref=sr_1_11?_mk_fr_FR=ÅMÅŽÕÑ& dchild=1&keywords=Fred+Evrard&qid=1612023803&sr=8-11

From the Square to the Compass – Reflections on Freemasonry and the Ageless Wisdom

https://www.amazon.fr/Square-Compass-Reflexions-Freemasonry-Ageless/dp/1793918813/ref=sr_1_14?_mk_fr_FR=ÅMÅŽÕÑ& dchild=1&keywords=Fred+Evrard&qid=1612023803&sr=8-14

Hakka Kung Fu – Martial Arts and culture of the Hakka People https://www.amazon.fr/Kung-Fu-Hakka-martiaux-culture/dp/1704788781/ref=sr_1_2?_mk_fr_FR=ÅMÅŽÕÑ&dchild=1&keywords=Fred+Evrard&qid=1612023803&sr=8-2

4 years around the world– Photo-album of our 4-year trip around the world

https://www.amazon.fr/Years-Around-World-Spirituality-Harley-Davidson/dp/B08BRGVPYF/ref=sr_1_9?_mk_fr_FR=ÅMÅŽÕÑ&dchild=1&keywords=Fred+Evrard&qid=1612023803&sr=8-9

Ancient & Accepted Scottish Rite

https://www.amazon.fr/Ancient-Accepted-Scottish-Rite-Freemasonry/dp/B08L411K93/ref=sr_1_6?_mk_fr_FR=ÅMÅŽÕÑ&dchild=1&keywords=Fred+Evrard&qid=1612023803&sr=8-6